Copyright 2023

All right reserved. No part of this book should be resproduce without express permission of the author.

Reproduction of all or any part of this book is punishable under relevant law.

Table of Contents

PREVIEW

Designed by behavioral psychologists, nutritionists and personal trainers, Noom's Weight program is aimed at helping you lose weight in the long run. It claims to focus on making tangible, sustainable lifestyle shifts rather than encouraging more extreme styles of eating (e.g., cutting out specific food groups or nutrients).

Unlike a traditional diet, Noom is a mobile health app subscription service that encourages people to make behavioral changes to live healthier.

Noom isn't new. It actually debuted in 2008 as a simple fitness and calorie tracker. But by 2016, the app had added a psychology and behavioral change component, user support groups and personal coaches.

Noom boasts a team of behavioral health experts who've researched oncology, diabetes prevention and management, hypertension and more to design a curriculum that gets to the root of weight loss struggles. Noom aims to help users focus on their mindset before they focus on meals. It is the company's philosophy that, "once you determine the things you're ready to work on, your mindset will help you form new neural connections over time to change your habits."

Today, losing weight the Noom way means examining eating behaviors, managing emotions related to food, practicing accountability and making lifestyle changes that can result in sustained weight loss.

NOOM DIET RECIPES

BREAKFAST

1.Easy Walnut Cake
Prep Time: 10 Minutes

Cook Time: 45 minutes

Servings: 15

Ingredients

- 1/2 cup butter (softened)
- 2 cups brown sugar (packed)
- 2 cups buttermilk
- 2 teaspoons baking soda
- 3 cups all-purpose flour
- 1 teaspoon vanilla extract

Nut Topping:

- 6 tablespoons butter (softened)
- 4 tablespoons milk
- 1 cup brown sugar (packed)
- 1/2 cup chopped pecans or walnuts

Instructions

1. Preheat the oven to 375 degrees. Spray a 9x13 baking pan with cooking spray.
2. In a large bowl, cream together the butter and sugar.
3. Add the buttermilk and baking soda. Mix well.

4. Add in the flour and vanilla. Mix until combined.
5. Pour the batter into the prepared pan. Bake at 375 degrees for 30 minutes or until the center bounces back when you touch it.
6. While the cake is baking, make the topping. In a bowl, combine the butter, milk, brown sugar and nuts. Mix well.
7. Spread this mixture all over the top of the warm cake.
8. Place under the broiler (turned to low) and bake for 1-3 minutes or until the nut topping is bubbling.
9. Remove from the oven and allow the cake to cool.
10. Serve warm alone, with whipped cream or with ice cream.

2. Thanksgiving Leftovers Casserole
Prep Time: 10 Minutes

Cook Time: 45 minutes

Servings: 15

Ingredients

- 4 cups turkey stuffing
- 2 cups chopped turkey
- 8 ounces swiss cheese shredded
- 12 large eggs
    - ounces cream of mushroom soup
- 1/4 cup whole milk
- 1 teaspoon poultry seasoning
- 1 teaspoon salt
- ½ teaspoon ground black pepper
- Fresh sage rosemary and thyme for topping, optional

Instructions

1. Preheat the oven to 350 degrees.
2. Spray a 9x13 baking pan with cooking spray.
3. Spread the turkey stuffing to cover the bottom of the prepared pan.
4. Sprinkle the chopped turkey over the stuffing.
5. Sprinkle the shredded cheese over the turkey.
6. Crack the 12 eggs into a large bowl.
7. Add the mushroom soup, milk, poultry seasoning, salt and pepper.
8. Whisk and mix well until the yolks are all broken up.
9. Pour the egg mixture over the cheese evenly.

10. Spray one side of a piece of aluminum foil with cooking spray.
11. Cover the baking pan, sprayed side down and seal the edges.
12. Bake in preheated oven for 30 minutes, then uncover and cook an additional 30-40 minutes or until the casserole is cooked through and the top is golden brown.
13. Top with optional herbs and serve warm.

3. Slow Cooker Casserole
Prep Time: 20 Minutes

Cook Time: 6hrs 2 minutes

Servings: 10

Ingredients

- 1 ½ cups diced ham
- ½ cup diced onion
- ½ cup diced bell peppers green, red or yellow
- 1 teaspoon ground pepper
- ½ teaspoon salt
- 2 cups frozen cubed potatoes
- 14 large eggs
- 1 cup half & half
- 12 ounces shredded sharp cheddar cheese divided
- Freshly snipped parsley for garnishing

Instructions

1. Place a disposable slow cooker liner inside and then up and over the sides of a slow cooker. Spray with cooking spray.
2. In a large bowl, combine the ham, onion, peppers, potatoes and seasonings. Mix well.
3. Pour this into the slow cooker and spread it evenly across the bottom.
4. In the same bowl, combine the eggs, half & half and 2/3 of the shredded cheese (8 ounces). Whisk until it is well mixed.

5. Pour the egg mixture evenly overtop the potatoes & ham.
6. Cover and cook on low for 6 hours.
7. Sprinkle the remaining cheese overtop the casserole, cover and cook for an additional 10 minutes to melt the cheese.
8. Garnish with fresh parsley if desired.

4. Gluten Free Casserole
Prep Time: 20 Minutes

Cook Time: 30 minutes

Servings: 10

Ingredients

White Sauce:

- 2 tablespoons butter
- 2 tablespoons tapioca flour or all-purpose flour
- 2 cups milk 2% or higher
- ½ teaspoon salt
- ½ teaspoon pepper
- 1/2 teaspoon ginger
- 1 teaspoon sage
- Dash of paprika

Other Ingredients:

- 30 ounces (about 7 cupfrozen shredded hash brown potatoes
- 6 large hard-boiled eggs peeled
- 2 cups shredded cheddar cheese
- 12 ounces bacon cooked and crumbled

Instructions

1. Pour the frozen shredded potatoes into a large bowl.
2. To make the white sauce, melt the butter in a saucepan over medium-low heat. Once the butter is

melted, add the tapioca flour and whisk until clumps are gone.

3. With the saucepan over medium heat, add 1 cup of milk and whisk until smooth.
4. Add the remaining milk and heat until slightly thickened, whisking often so the milk does not scorch. With tapioca flour, this only took 3-4 minutes. (If you use all-purpose flour, it will take longer.)
5. Remove from the heat and stir in salt, pepper, ginger, sage and paprika. Pour the white sauce over the shredded potatoes, mix and set aside.
6. Heat the oven to 375 degrees.
7. Spray a 9x13 baking pan with cooking spray.
8. Pour and spread half of the shredded potatoes on bottom of the baking pan.
9. Slice each hardboiled egg lengthwise, making 4 slices for each egg, equaling 24 slices.
10. Lay the egg slices down flat, covering the potatoes.
11. Pour and spread the remaining potato mixture over the eggs.
12. Sprinkle the cheese overtop the potatoes.
13. Then sprinkle the cooked & crumbled bacon over the cheese.
14. Bake at 375 for 30 minutes.

5. Strawberry Muffins
Prep Time: 20 Minutes

Cook Time: 20 minutes

Servings: 12

Ingredients

For The Muffins:

- 3/4 cup granulated sugar 150 grams
- 1/2 cup 2% milk 4 ounces
- 1/2 cup canola oil 4 ounces
- 1 large egg
- 1 teaspoon vanilla extract 5 grams
- 1 teaspoon almond extract 5 grams
- 2 cups all-purpose flour 260 grams
- 1 teaspoon baking powder 3 grams
- 1/2 teaspoon baking soda 2 grams
- 1/2 teaspoon salt 3 grams
- 2 cups finely diced fresh strawberries 315 grams

For The Crumble:

- 1/2 cup granulated sugar 100 grams
- 1/2 cup all-purpose flour 65 grams
- 3 tablespoons salted butter softened

For The Glaze:

- 1 cup powdered sugar 130 grams
- 1 tablespoon salted butter melted
- 1/4 teaspoon almond extract
- 3 tablespoons finely diced strawberries

- 1-2 tablespoons heavy cream optional, if needed

Instructions

1. Preheat the oven to 425°F. Spray a 12-cup muffin pan with Baker's Joy baking spray (choose a baking spray with flour for best results).
2. In a large bowl, whisk together the sugar, milk, oil, egg, vanilla and almond extract.
3. In a separate medium bowl, combine the flour, baking powder, baking soda and salt.
4. Add the flour mixture to the wet ingredients and stir until just combined. Do not overmix.
5. Fold the strawberries gently into the batter.
6. Spoon the batter into the 12 muffin cups, dividing the batter evenly.
7. Make the crumble by mixing together the flour, sugar and butter in a small bowl. Don't overmix this. It's ok if it is a little floury. This mixture will be crumbly.
8. Divide the crumbs between the 12 muffins, sprinkling the crumbs on top of the batter.
9. Bake at 425°F for 5 minutes, then lower the oven temperature (without opening the oven) to 350°F and bake for an additional 16-18 minutes. A toothpick inserted in the center of the muffin should come out clean.
10. Allow the muffins to cool for about 3 minutes in the pan, then remove the muffins and place them on a wire rack to cool completely.
11. Store at room temperature in an airtight container for up to 24 hours, then refrigerate for up to 3 more days.

6. Strawberry Rolls
Prep Time: 30 Minutes

Cook Time: 25 minutes

Servings: 12

Ingredients

For The Dough:

- 1 cup warm milk (about 115 degrees F)
- 2 1/4 teaspoons instant dry yeast I like Red Star Platinum Baking Yeast
- 2 large eggs (at room temperature)
- 1/2 cup salted butter (Melted, but make sure it isn't super hot. Just barely melted, or even softened, is fine.)
- 4 1/2 cups all-purpose flour (divided)
- 1 teaspoon salt
- 1/2 cup granulated sugar

For The Filling:

- 6 ounces cream cheese (room temperature)
- 1/3 cup strawberry jam
- 2 cups diced strawberries

For The Cream Bath:

- 1/2 cup heavy cream (for pouring over the risen rolls)

For The Frosting:

- 2 cups powdered sugar
- 1/4 teaspoon salt

- 1/2 teaspoon vanilla extract (or almond)
- 2 ounces cream cheese softened
- 1/2 cup diced strawberries

Instructions

1. Pour the warm milk in the bowl of a stand mixer and sprinkle the yeast overtop.
2. Add the eggs, butter, salt and sugar.
3. Add in 4 cups (save the other ½ cup and add only if you need it) of flour and mix using the beater blade just until the ingredients are barely combined. Allow the mixture to rest for 5 minutes so the flour has time to soak up the liquids.
4. Scrape the dough off the beater blade and remove it. Attach the dough hook.
5. Beat the dough on medium speed, adding in up to ½ cup more flour if needed to form a dough. Knead for 5-7 minutes or until the dough is elastic and smooth. The dough should be tacky and will still be sticking to the sides of the bowl. That's ok! Don't be tempted to add more flour at this point. We generally add about 4 ½ cups, but start with 4 cups.
6. Spray a large bowl with cooking spray.
7. Use a rubber spatula to remove the dough from the mixer bowl and place it in the greased large bowl.
8. Cover the bowl with a towel or wax paper.
9. Set the bowl in a warm place and allow the dough to rise until double. I like to turn on the oven to the lowest setting for 1-2 minutes. Then turn off the oven and place the dough to rise in there. It normally takes about 30 minutes for the dough to rise. Do not allow

the dough to rise too much or your cinnamon rolls will be airy.

10. While the dough is rising, prepare the filling. In a medium bowl, use a hand mixer to beat the cream cheese and strawberry jam until smooth and creamy. Set aside.
11. Sprinkle a pastry mat with flour. Turn out the dough onto the lightly floured work surface and sprinkle the top of the dough with additional flour.
12. Flour a rolling pin and roll the dough to about a 24×15″ rectangle. (the size of the rectangle can vary...it does not have to be exact!)
13. Use a rubber spatula to smooth the cream cheese filling over the whole dough rectangle. Then sprinkle the diced strawberries evenly over the filling.
14. Starting on the long end, roll the dough up tightly jelly roll style.
15. Cut into 12 slices and place in a greased 10×15″ baking pan.
16. Cover the pan and allow the rolls to rise for 20 minutes or until nearly double.
17. Preheat the oven to 375 degrees.
18. Warm the heavy cream until the chill is off. Don't make it hot...you just don't want it cold. It should be warm to the touch.
19. Once the rolls have risen, pour the heavy cream over the top of the rolls, allowing it to soak down in and around the rolls.
20. Bake at 375 degrees for 22-25 minutes, until the rolls are lightly golden brown and the center rolls are cooked through. Note...the time will vary based on how big the rolls are, what type of pan, how close the rolls are packed, etc. They could take up to 25-27 minutes. Check the rolls at 20 minutes. If they are

getting too browned, cover loosely with foil for the remaining baking time.

21. While the rolls are cooling, prepare the cream cheese frosting.
22. In a large bowl, combine the powdered sugar, salt, vanilla extract, softened cream cheese and diced strawberries using a hand mixer. At first it won't seem like the glaze is coming together, but don't be tempted to add any liquid. Allow the mix to sit for a minute or just keep mixing on low speed. The strawberries will release juices and the frosting will eventually become spreadable. If for some reason yours is not after you've given it several minutes, add a tablespoon of heavy cream.
23. Spread the frosting over the cooled rolls.
24. Store in an airtight container in the refrigerator.

7. Home Fried Potatoes
Prep Time: 15 Minutes

Cook Time: 15 minutes

Servings: 4

Ingredients

- 2 pounds Russet potatoes
- 3 tablespoons vegetable oil peanut oil or coconut oil
- 1 teaspoon salt
- 1/2 teaspoon black pepper
- 1/2 teaspoon garlic powder
- 1/2 teaspoon onion powder

Instructions

1. Wash the potatoes and cut into 1-inch cubes.
2. Place the cubes in a large bowl and cover with water. Allow them to sit for 30 minutes.
3. Drain the water off the potatoes and rinse the potatoes.
4. Pour 6 cups of water in a large pot and add the potatoes.
5. Heat the potatoes until boiling, then allow to boil 5 minutes or until mostly soft. The exact timing will depend on how big the pieces of potato are. The need to be tender, but they'll cook a little longer in the pan.
6. Drain the potatoes and let them steam dry to evaporate the moisture.
7. Heat 3 tablespoons of oil in a nonstick large skillet over medium high heat.

8. Add the potatoes, then sprinkle the seasoning on top.
9. Cook and stir the potatoes for about 10-15 minutes until they are golden brown. If the skillet is not non-stick, you may have to add more oil so that they don't stick to the bottom. With non-stick pans, you can use less oil, but don't scrimp on the oil if you want the potatoes to be golden brown.
10. Serve the potatoes right away. Store any leftovers in the refrigerator in an airtight container for up to 3 days.

8. Peanut Butter Streusel Chocolate Chip Pancakes
Prep Time: 15 Minutes

Cook Time: 15 minutes

Servings: 10

Ingredients

- 1 1/3 cups all-purpose flour
- 3 teaspoons baking powder aluminum free
- 3/4 teaspoon salt
- 1 1/4 cups 2% milk
- 1 large egg
- 3 tablespoons canola oil
- 2 tablespoons granulated sugar
- 1/2 cup chocolate chips

Streusel:

- 1/2 cup plus 1 tablespoon all-purpose flour
- 1/2 cup packed brown sugar
- 1/4 cup salted butter softened
- 3 tablespoons peanut butter
- 1/2 cup mini chocolate chips

Instructions

1. To Prevent Salmonella Or Other Harmful Bacteria, Cook The Raw Flour Before Making The Streusel.
2. Preheat the oven to 350°F. Line a small baking pan with parchment paper. Sprinkle the ½ cup plus 1

tablespoon of flour onto the baking sheet. Bake flour for 5 minutes. Then remove and cool the flour.

For The Pancakes:

1. In a medium bowl, whisk together the flour, baking powder and salt. Set aside.
2. In another larger bowl, whisk together the milk, egg, oil and sugar.
3. Add the dry ingredients to the wet ingredients and mix gently just until combined. Do not over mix.
4. Gently fold in the chocolate chips.
5. Let the batter rest for 15 minutes. This will result in a fluffier, tender pancake.
6. Lightly grease a skillet with cooking spray, butter, or oil. My favorite choice is melted butter. Heat over medium low heat.
7. Ladle about ⅓ cup of the pancake batter onto the preheated skillet. Allow the pancake to cook until it is bubbly on top, then turn and finish by cooking on the other side until the pancake is cooked through.

Make The Streusel:

1. Combine the flour, sugar, softened butter, peanut butter and chocolate chips in a small bowl until crumbly.
2. Top the pancakes with butter, streusel and your favorite maple syrup or whipped cream.
3. Store any leftovers in an airtight container in the fridge.

9. Strawberry Scones

Prep Time: 20 Minutes

Cook Time: 14 minutes

Servings: 8

Ingredients

- 2 1/4 cups all-purpose flour 293 grams
- 1 1/4 teaspoons baking soda 6 grams
- 2 teaspoons cream of tartar 7 grams
- 2 tablespoons granulated sugar 24 grams
- dash salt
- 1/2 cup plus 1 tablespoon cold salted butter 9 tablespoons
- 1 large beaten egg
- 3/4 cup thick buttermilk 6 ounces
- 1 1/2 cups chopped strawberries 232 grams

Streusel:

- 1/4 cup granulated sugar 50 grams
- 1/4 cup all-purpose flour 33 grams
- 1 1/2 tablespoons salted butter

Glaze:

- 1 cup powdered sugar 130 grams
- 3 tablespoons melted butter
- 1/2 teaspoon vanilla extract
- 1-2 tablespoons heavy cream or milk if needed to thin glaze

Instructions

1. Refrigerate or freeze a glass bowl for 5 minutes to get it cold.
2. Preheat the oven to 425°F. Line a baking sheet with parchment paper.
3. In the refrigerated bowl, add the flour, baking soda, cream of tartar, sugar and salt. Whisk well.
4. Cut the cold butter into small cubes and add to the flour mixture. Using a pastry cutter, cut the butter in with the flour mixture until the butter is mostly mixed in. You can also use your fingers to "snap" the butter between your fingers to break it up. It is okay if there are small pieces of butter.
5. Make a well in the flour, in the center of the bowl. Add the egg and buttermilk to the well. Using a wooden spoon, mix the wet ingredients into the dry ingredients and mix just until barely combined.
6. Add the diced strawberries and fold together just 2-3 times until they are evenly distributed. Do not over mix.
7. Sprinkle flour on top a pastry mat Turn the dough out onto the floured surface. Sprinkle a little more flour on top of the dough, then shape it into a disk that is about 1 1/4" thick.
8. In a small bowl, combine the ingredients for the streusel. Cut the butter into the sugar and flour until it is coarse crumbs. Sprinkle the streusel over the dough circle and pat it down gently to press it in.
9. Use a sharp knife or dough cutter to cut the disk into 8 triangles, as if you were cutting a pie. Place the scones on the prepared baking pan. Sprinkle any streusel that may have fallen off back on the top of the scones.

10. Refrigerate or freeze the sheet of scones for 10-15
    minutes. (10 in the freezer, 15 in the fridge)
11. Bake immediately for 12-14 minutes. Allow the scones
    to cool for 10 minutes and prepare the glaze.
12. In a small bowl, melt the 3 tablespoons of butter. Add
    in the powdered sugar and vanilla. Mix well. If
    needed, add 1-2 tablespoons of cream in order to
    easily spoon the glaze over the scones.
13. Glaze the top of the scones.
14. Store in an airtight container in the fridge for up to 3
    days.

10. Funfetti Pancakes from a Cake Mix
Prep Time: 10 Minutes

Cook Time: 15 minutes

Servings: 11

Ingredients

- 1 1/3 cups all-purpose flour
- 2 teaspoons baking powder
- 2 tablespoons granulated sugar
- 1/2 teaspoon salt
- 1 box Pillsbury Funfetti cake mix (15.25 ounces)
- 1/3 cup canola oil
- 3 large eggs
- 2 1/3 cups 2% milk
- 1/3 cup sprinkles

Frosting:

- 1 cup powdered sugar
- 2 tablespoons salted butter softened
- 2 tablespoons half & half cream
- 1/2 teaspoon vanilla extract or almond extract

Instructions

1. In a large mixing bowl, combine the flour, baking powder, sugar, salt and cake mix. Set aside.
2. In another small bowl, whisk together the oil, eggs and milk.

3. Add the wet ingredients into the dry ingredients and mix just until combined. Fold in the sprinkles. Batter will be thick. (If you'd like thinner pancakes, you can add a bit more milk.)
4. Heat a griddle to about 250-275 degrees Fahrenheit (low heat so the pancakes do not burn). Spray the griddle with cooking spray.
5. Ladle the pancake batter onto the hot pan and cook the pancakes for about 1-2 minutes or until bubbles start forming in the batter. Flip the pancake and cook for an additional minute or until cooked through.
6. This recipes makes about 22 5″ pancakes.

For The Frosting

1. In a small bowl, stir together the powdered sugar, softened butter, cream and vanilla. This frosting will be at a spreadable consistency.
2. If you'd like to drizzle the frosting, microwave the frosting for about 10 seconds and stir, then drizzle over the pancakes.
3. Double the frosting recipe, if desired.
4. Drizzle the glaze overtop the pancakes.
5. Store any leftovers in an airtight container in the fridge for up to 4 days.

LUNCH

11.Ohio Shredded Chicken Sandwiches
Prep Time: 5 Minutes

Cook Time: 4hrs 2 minutes

Servings: 10

Ingredients

- 3 pounds boneless skinless chicken breasts
- 2 cans condensed cream of chicken soup (10.75 ounces each)
- 1 box chicken flavored Stove Top Stuffing (6 ounces)
- chicken broth (to thin only if the mixture seems to thick)

Instructions

1. Place the chicken breasts in the slow cooker.
2. Pour the condensed soup overtop.
3. Cover and cook on low for 3-4 hours or until the chicken is shreddable.
4. Shred the chicken, then add the stuffing mix.
5. Mix well, cover and cook for 15-20 minutes or until the bread crumbs are moistened.
6. If you'd like the mixture thinner, add a little bit of chicken broth until it is the consistency you'd like.
7. Serve on hamburger buns.

12. Mexican Meatloaf Sandwiches
Prep Time: 10 Minutes

Cook Time: 55 minutes

Servings: 8

Ingredients

For The Meatloaf

- 2 pounds ground chuck (85% lean)
- 2 large eggs
- 1/2 cup quick cooking oats
- 1/3 cup chopped green pepper
- 1/4 cup chopped red onion
- 1 tablespoon paprika
- 1 tablespoon chili powder
- 1/2 tablespoon cumin
- 1/2 tablespoon oregano
- 1/2 teaspoon dry mustard
- 1/4 teaspoon black pepper
- 1/4 teaspoon salt
- 1 1/2 cups shredded cheddar cheese

Sandwich Ingredients

Sponsored Content

- Sponsored Video by nescafe.com
- By nescafe.com
- 16 slices bread
- 8 slices sliced colby cheese
- 2 cups fresh salsa

Instructions

1. Preheat the oven to 350 degrees Fahrenheit. Line a 9×5" baking pan with parchment paper. (Or spray with cooking spray.)
2. Combine all of the meatloaf ingredients in a large bowl. Mix well.
3. Press the beef mixture into the loaf pan.
4. Bake for 55-60 minutes, or until the internal temperature reads 165 degrees.
5. Allow the meatloaf to rest for 5 minutes, then slice and serve.
6. To make the sandwiches, place a slice of meatloaf on a piece of bread. Top with cheese and fresh salsa. Place a second piece of bread on the top.
7. Serve immediately.

13. Scotcheroo Bars
Prep Time: 15 Minutes

Cook Time: 5 minutes

Servings: 20

Ingredients

- 1 cup light corn syrup
- 1 cup sugar
- 1 cup creamy peanut butter
- 6 cups Kellogg's Rice Krispies cereal
- 1 1/2 cups semi-sweet chocolate chips
- 1 1/2 cups butterscotch chips
- 1 tablespoon salted butter room temperature

Instructions

1. Line a 9×13 baking pan with parchment paper or foil, then spray lightly with cooking spray.
2. Place the corn syrup and the sugar in a saucepan. Cook and stir over medium heat until sugar dissolves. You don't want to let the mixture boil. If you see a sign of the mixture boiling, remove it immediately from the heat. 1 cup light corn syrup, 1 cup sugar
3. Stir the peanut butter into the corn syrup mixture and mix until smooth. 1 cup creamy peanut butter
4. Add the cereal and stir until well coated. Press the mixture lightly into the pan. Don't press tightly or the bars might be too hard. Just make sure the mix is even. 6 cups Kellogg's Rice Krispies cereal

5. In a microwave safe bowl, melt chocolate and butterscotch chips together in 30-second intervals, stirring between each interval until the chocolate mixture is smooth. 1 ½ cups semi-sweet chocolate chips, 1 ½ cups butterscotch chips
6. Add the butter to the chocolate and mix until smooth and even. 1 tablespoon salted butter
7. Spread evenly over cereal mixture.
8. Then lastly, sprinkle with sea salt if you'd like.
9. Let the chocolate set, then cut into squares.
10. Store in an airtight container at room temperature.
11. To freeze, wrap the scotcheroo bars individually in plastic wrap, then place in the freezer. Pull them out to thaw as you'd like.

14. Pepperoni Pizza Sliders
Prep Time: 10 Minutes

Cook Time: 25 minutes

Servings: 12

Ingredients

- 1/2 cup Challenge Butter salted butter melted
- 1 tablespoon sesame seeds
- 1 teaspoon Italian seasoning
- 2 tablespoons grated Parmesan
- 1/2 teaspoon crushed red pepper flakes
- 1 teaspoon garlic powder
- 12 Hawaiian dinner rolls 18 ounces
- 12 slices sliced provolone cheese 8 ounces
- 8 slices large thinly sliced pepperoni 3 ounces
- 6 slices thinly sliced Genoa hard salami 2 ounces
- 6 slices thinly sliced deli ham 2 ounces
- 1 tablespoon freshly snipped parsley
- ¾ cup pizza sauce for serving

Instructions

1. Preheat oven to 350 degrees Fahrenheit.
2. Line a baking sheet with parchment paper or foil. Spray very lightly with cooking spray.
3. In a bowl, mix together butter, sesame seeds, Italian seasoning, parmesan, red pepper flakes and garlic powder.

4. Use a large serrated knife to slice the rolls in half, separating the tops from the bottoms. Place the bottom of the rolls onto the prepared baking pan.
5. Brush ⅓ of the butter mixture onto the bottom buns.
6. Layer on half of the cheese, then all of the pepperoni, salami, the remaining cheese and then the ham.
7. Place the tops of the rolls onto the sandwiches.
8. Brush another ⅓ of the butter mixture evenly over the rolls.
9. Cover the rolls loosely with foil.
10. Bake in the preheated oven until the rolls are lightly browned and the cheese has melted, about 25 minutes.
11. Remove the foil and bake for an additional 3-5 minutes or until lightly browned and cheese is melted.
12. Add the freshly snipped parsley to the leftover butter.
13. Brush the remaining butter sauce over the rolls.
14. Slice into individual rolls through the ham and cheese layers to serve immediately with sauce on the side.

Prep Time: 20 Minutes

Cook Time: 00 minutes

Servings: 8

Ingredients

- 2 cups chopped Roma tomatoes
- 1 cup chopped red onion
- 1 small jalapeno pepper chopped
- 1/4 cup chopped poblano pepper
- 1 1/2 cup fresh corn cut off the cob
- 1/4 cup fresh cilantro chopped
- 2 teaspoons minced garlic
- 1/4 teaspoon pepper
- 1/2 teaspoon salt
- 1/4 cup lime juice
- 1 avocado cut into small pieces

Instructions

1. Combine all of the ingredients together in a bowl and stir gently to combine.
2. Serve immediately.
3. Store any leftovers in an airtight container in the refrigerator.

16. Homemade Italian Meatballs

Prep Time: 20 Minutes

Cook Time: 35 minutes

Servings: 10

Ingredients

- 2 pounds lean ground beef
- 3/4 pound ground Italian sausage
- 4 large eggs
- 1 cup Parmesan cheese
- 1/2 cup Italian bread crumbs
- 1 1/2 tablespoons dried parsley
- 1/2 teaspoon dried basil
- 1 teaspoon garlic salt
- 1/4 teaspoon black pepper

Instructions

1. In a large bowl, mix all of the ingredients together.
2. Roll into 1 1/2" balls and place them closely together in 9×13 pans that have been sprayed with cooking spray. **You can place a wire rack on the baking sheet and bake the meatballs on the rack so that the fat drips down if you'd like.
3. Bake at 350 degrees for 35 minutes, or until the meatballs are cooked through.
4. Serve the meatballs immediately with sauce and spaghetti, put them in the slow cooker along with sauce to have them simmer, or freeze the meatballs in Ziploc bags to use another time.

5. If you freeze the meatballs, allow them to cool completely before packaging them.

17. Paleo Shepherd's Pie
Prep Time: 30 Minutes

Cook Time: 30 minutes

Servings: 6

Ingredients

- 5 large Russet potatoes peeled and cut into chunks (2 pounds)
- 1/4 cup salted butter ghee or coconut oil
- 1/2 cup almond milk
- salt and pepper to taste

Sauce:

- 1/2 cup petite diced tomatoes
- 3/4 cup beef stock
- 1 teaspoon basil
- 2 teaspoons minced garlic
- 1 teaspoon Italian seasoning
- 1/2 teaspoon salt
- 2 teaspoons tapioca starch or corn starch

Filling:

- 1 1/3 pound ground beef
- 1 small onion chopped (½ cup)
- 1 cup chopped carrots
- 1 cup zucchini peeled and chopped
- 1 cup frozen peas
- 1 cup finely chopped kale

Instructions

1. In a large saucepan, boil the potatoes until they are tender (about 10 minutes). Mash the potatoes and cream them together with the butter, milk, salt and pepper until they are fluffy. Set aside.
2. Place all of the sauce ingredients into a blender and blend until smooth. Set aside.
3. Brown the ground beef and onions in a large skillet or saucepan. Drain the fat off the meat.
4. Add the sauce and chopped vegetables to the skillet. Cover the skillet and allow the meat and veggies to simmer for 10-15 minutes until the veggies start getting tender. Don't allow them to cook all the way through since they will continue to cook in the oven.
5. Preheat the oven to 350 degrees Fahrenheit. Transfer the meat and veggies to a 9×13 pan or a deep dish 9×9 casserole pan. Top the meat mixture with the mashed potatoes and spread out evenly. Bake for 25-30 minutes or until heated through and bubbly around the edges.
6. Serve warm.

18. Kale Tomato Skillet Lasagna
Prep Time: 15 Minutes

Cook Time: 5 minutes

Servings: 4

Ingredients

- 1 tablespoon olive oil
- 1/2 cup chopped onion
- 2 garlic cloves minced
- 1 pound ground beef
- 2 cups kale chopped
- 2 tomatoes diced
- 2 teaspoons oregano
- 6 ounces penne pasta
- 6 ounces fresh mozzarella cheese torn into small pieces

Instructions

1. Sauté olive oil, onion and garlic over medium low heat until onions are tender.
2. Add ground beef to skillet and cook until done, drain grease and set ground beef aside.
3. While the beef is browning, bring a pot of water to a boil and cook pasta according to package instructions.
4. Cook kale in skillet until wilted, add a splash or two of water if it's not wilting.
5. Add tomatoes to kale in skillet and cook until tomatoes begin to break down. Add ¼ cup of water if needed to help tomatoes cook.

6. Add in oregano and return ground beef to the pan.
7. Mix in cooked pasta and half of the mozzarella cheese.
8. Mix everything together well in the skillet and top with remaining mozzarella cheese.
9. Heat the oven to broil and place in oven for 3-5 minutes, or until cheese is melted.

19. Grilled Lemon Lime Pepper Chicken
Prep Time: 20 Minutes

Cook Time: 20 minutes

Servings: 6

Ingredients

- 2 pounds boneless skinless chicken breasts about 6 small pieces
- 1 cup olive oil
- 1/3 cup lemon juice
- 1/3 cup lime juice
- 2 teaspoons minced garlic
- 1 medium onion diced
- 1/2 teaspoon pepper
- 1/2 teaspoon salt

Instructions

1. Mix together olive oil, lemon & lime juice, garlic, salt, pepper and onion.
2. Put chicken in a Ziploc bag and pour marinade over it. Allow to marinate overnight in the refrigerator.
3. Place chicken on preheated grill (400 degrees) and cook for about 10 minutes on each side, or until the chicken is no longer pink.
4. Allow the chicken to rest for 3-5 minutes, then serve.
5. Store any leftovers in the refrigerator in an airtight container for up to 3 days.

20. Strawberry Spinach Salad
Prep Time: 10 Minutes

Cook Time: 00 minutes

Servings: 3

Ingredients

- 9 ounces baby spinach and lettuce mix
- 5-6 medium strawberries sliced
- 1/2 medium red onion sliced
- 4 ounces feta cheese
- 1/2 cup sliced almonds

Poppyseed Dressing

- 1/2 cup olive oil
- 1/4 cup apple cider vinegar
- 5 tablespoons Swerve sweetner (or sugar of your choice)
- 1/8 teaspoon salt
- 1 tablespoon poppy seeds
- 2 drops of liquid stevia (optional, to taste)

Instructions

For The Salad:

1. Wash strawberries. Slice them and set aside.
2. Place the lettuce mixture into a large bowl.
3. Slice onion thinly and add to lettuce.
4. Crumble cheese and sprinkle over salad.
5. Add strawberries and almonds to the mixture.

For The Dressing:

1. Add all ingredients to a mason jar.
2. Shake together to incorporate.

Make The Salad:

1. Just before serving, drizzle the desired amount of poppyseed dressing over the salad and toss to coat.

DINNER

21. No Knead Jalapeño Cheese Bread
Prep Time: 10 Minutes

Cook Time: 40 minutes

Servings: 10

Ingredients

- 3 1/4 cups bread flour (or up to ½ cup more if needed) 393 grams
- 1 teaspoon salt 8 grams
- 1 teaspoon instant yeast 5 grams
- 2 jalapeno peppers 55-65 grams each
- 1 teaspoon minced garlic 7 grams
- 2 cups shredded sharp cheddar cheese 184 grams
- 1 1/3 cups warm water about 95-100°F

Instructions

Make The Dough:

2. In a large mixing bowl, whisk together the flour and salt.
3. Add in the yeast and whisk again.
4. Finely dice 1 jalapeno pepper.
5. Add the diced pepper, minced garlic and shredded cheese to the flour mixture. Mix until combined.
6. Stir in water, mixing thoroughly until you have a smooth uniform dough. The dough will be sticky, but that's what you want. If it isn't coming together in a

ball, add up to ½ cup more flour, but the dough should be sticky to the touch.

7. Cover tightly with plastic wrap and let sit at room temperature for 4-6 hours, or until the dough has risen to nearly double the size.

8. Use a rubber spatula to fold the dough together several times. Form into a ball. Cover and allow the dough to rest for another 30-60 minutes while the oven is preheating.

Bake The Bread:

1. Preheat the oven to 450°F.
2. Use a rubber spatula to scrape dough onto a piece of parchment paper.
3. Press sliced jalapeno peppers into the top of the dough ball.
4. Place the dough ball (with parchment paper) into a Dutch oven. Place the Dutch oven cover on.
5. Turn the oven down to 425° Fahrenheit. Then bake the bread in the covered Dutch oven for 30 minutes.
6. Remove the lid, remove the parchment paper with loaf on it and place it right on the oven rack. Continue to bake for another 10 minutes or until the bread is golden brown.
7. Allow the bread to rest for at least 10 minutes before slicing and serving with Zoup! Good, Really Good ® Spicy Chicken 'Chilada TM Soup.

22.Easy Cheeseburger Soup
Prep Time: 10 Minutes

Cook Time: 25 minutes

Servings: 8

Ingredients

- 1 pound lean ground beef
- ¾ cup chopped onion
- ¾ cup shredded carrots
- ¾ cup chopped celery
- 2 teaspoons minced garlic
- 1 teaspoon dried basil
- 1 teaspoon dried parsley
- ½ teaspoon ground mustard
- ½ teaspoon salt
- ½ teaspoon black pepper
- ¼ teaspoon paprika
- 4 cups cubed potatoes peeled
- 4 cups chicken broth or chicken stock
- 2 tablespoons cornstarch
- 1 can evaporated milk 12 ounces
- 3 cups shredded Cheddar cheese
- ¼ cup sour cream optional

Instructions

1. Add ground beef, onion, carrots, and celery to a large dutch oven over medium heat. Cook and stir until beef is browned and crumbled. Drain off any fat.

2. Add in all of the seasonings.
3. Then add the potatoes and stock. and bring to a boil; reduce heat to low and simmer until potatoes are tender, 15-20 minutes.
4. Whisk the cornstarch into the evaporated milk until smooth.
5. Then drizzle the milk slowly into the soup, stirring constantly.
6. With the burner still on low, continue to cook and stir while the soup thickens. Add the cheese, a handful at a time, stirring between each addition.
7. Stir in the sour cream if you'd like to add it.
8. Then serve in bowls and garnish with homemade croutons and freshly snipped parsley.
9. Store any leftovers in an airtight container in the fridge for up to 4 days.

23. Sizzling Steak Fajitas
Prep Time: 15 Minutes

Cook Time: 20 minutes

Servings: 6

Ingredients

- 1 1/2 pounds flank steak
- 4 tablespoons fajita seasoning
- 2 tablespoons olive oil
- 1 large red onion
- 1 red bell pepper
- 1 green bell pepper
- salt and pepper (to taste)

Optional Toppings:

- flour tortillas
- shredded cheddar cheese
- sour cream
- guacamole

Instructions

1. Remove the flank steak from the refrigerator 30 minutes before grilling.
2. Rub the fajita seasoning into both sides of the steak and allow it to rest for 30 minutes.
3. Heat a grill to 450°F.
4. Place the steak on the grill and cook for 4-6 minutes on each side, until the internal temperature reaches the desired doneness.

5. Remove the steak from the grill and allow it to rest for 5 minutes before slicing.
6. Heat the oven to 400°F. Place the cast iron fajita skillets into the oven for at least 20 minutes in order to get a good sizzle.
7. While the fajita pans are heating, heat the oil in a skillet on the stovetop over medium heat.
8. Slice the onions and peppers into thin slices.
9. Add the vegetable slices to the hot oil and fry until they are tender, yet still crisp. Season with salt and pepper, to taste.
10. While the vegetables are cooking, slice the steak down the middle (if it is a wide steak), then slice it against the grain the size steak slices you'd like.
11. When the vegetables and fajita skillets are ready, remove the cast iron skillets from the oven adn quickly arrange the beef and peppers on it. It will immediately start to sizzle.
12. Serve the sizzling skillets with warm tortillas and other fajita toppings of your choice.

24. Broccoli Cheddar Soup
Prep Time: 10 Minutes

Cook Time: 25 minutes

Servings: 8

Ingredients

- ¼ cup salted butter
- ½ cup diced onion
- 1 teaspoon minced garlic
- ¼ cup all-purpose flour
- 3 cups chicken stock
- 1 cup 2% milk warmed
- 1 cup heavy cream warmed
- 1 teaspoon dijon mustard
- 1 teaspoon salt
- ¼ teaspoon white pepper
- dash hot pepper sauce
- 3 cups broccoli florets
- 1 cup shredded carrots
- 3 cups freshly shredded sharp cheddar cheese

Instructions

1. In a dutch oven or large soup pot, melt the butter over medium-high heat.
2. Saute the onion and garlic in the butter for 2-3 minutes.
3. Add the flour and quickly whisk.

4. Pour in one cup of the chicken stock, and whisk until the mixture is smooth.
5. Add the remaining 2 cups of chicken stock and whisk again.
6. Add in the milk, heavy cream, dijon mustard, pepper and hot sauce. Whisk constantly over medium heat for about 3-5 minutes until the mixture starts to steam and almost comes to a boil. Then turn the stovetop medium-low heat.
7. Add in the broccoli and shredded carrots. Cook, stirring often, for about 15-20 minutes until the broccoli is tender. The exact timing will depend on the size of the broccoli florets.
8. If you'd like a smoother soup, use an immersion blender to purée about one third to half of the soup. Or you can leave the soup with the larger vegetable pieces.
9. Once the broccoli is tender, turn the heat to low and add in the shredded cheddar cheese, about ¼ cup at a time, stirring so that the cheese melts between each addition.
10. Serve immediately.

25. Vegetarian Pecan Tomato Pasta

Prep Time: 10 Minutes

Cook Time: 18 minutes

Servings: 8

Ingredients

- 1 pound gemelli pasta
- ½ cup unsalted pecans
- 2 tablespoons oil from sundried tomatoes or olive oil
- ¼ cup sun dried tomatoes from can or jar
- 2 heirloom tomatoes diced
- 1 shallot diced
- 2 garlic cloves minced
- 1 teaspoon dried oregano
- ½ teaspoon red pepper flakes
- 1 ½ cup kale chopped
- 2 ½ tablespoons fresh basil chopped
- 2 tablespoons fresh parsley chopped
- ½ teaspoon salt
- ½ teaspoon pepper

Instructions

1. Boil and drain pasta according to the package instructions. Cook to al dente.
2. While the pasta is cooking, prepare the next steps.
3. Add pecans to a food processor and pulse to break apart into small pieces.

4. Add sun dried tomato oil, chopped heirloom tomatoes, chopped sun dried tomatoes, minced shallot, minced garlic, oregano and red pepper flakes to a deep frying pan. Sauté for 5 minutes.
5. Stir in the kale and pecans. Cook until wilted for 5 minutes.
6. Add noodles, ½ the basil and parsley. Stir in the salt and pepper and cook for 5 minutes to heat through.
7. Garnish with remaining basil and parsley and serve immediately.
8. Store any leftovers in an airtight container in the fridge for up to 4 days.

26. How to Cook a Boston Butt
Prep Time: 5 Minutes

Cook Time: 8hrs 3 minutes

Servings: 20

Ingredients

- 7-8 pounds Boston Butt or pork shoulder

For The Pulled Pork Rub:

- 1/2 cup smoked paprika
- 1/3 cup dark brown sugar
- 1/4 cup salt
- 1/4 cup garlic powder
- 2 tablespoons black pepper
- 2 tablespoons chili powder
- 2 tablespoons onion powder
- 2 tablespoons chipotle chili pepper
- 1 tablespoon cayenne pepper
- 1 tablespoon cumin
- 1 tablespoon dry mustard

Instructions

1. Preheat the oven to 450°F.
2. Mix all of the spices together in a bowl.
3. Rub the spice mix on all sides of the pork butt.
4. Place the pork butt fat side up in a roasting pan with a rack.
5. Bake for 30 minutes at 450°F. Then, without opening the oven, reduce the oven temperature to 250°F. Bake

for 7-8 hours or until the internal temperature of the pork reaches 195-200°F.
6. Take the pork out of the oven, cover it with aluminum foil and allow it to rest for 15 minutes.
7. Then use meat forks to shred the meat.
8. Save some of the juices from the pork to store the leftovers in. It helps keep the pork juicy.
9. Store any leftover pork in an airtight container for up to 3 days.
10. Freeze any leftovers for up to 6 weeks.

27. Irish Soda Bread
Prep Time: 15 Minutes

Cook Time: 50 minutes

Servings: 10

Ingredients

For The Bread:

- 4 cups all-purpose flour 520 grams
- 1 1/2 teaspoons baking soda
- ½ teaspoon salt
- 2 tablespoons granulated sugar
- ¾ cup cold salted butter cut into tablespoons, 6 ounces
- 1 ⅓ cups buttermilk

For Topping:

- 1 tablespoon buttermilk
- 1 tablespoon melted butter

Instructions

1. Preheat the oven to 375°F. Place a piece of parchment paper into a baking pan or skillet.
2. Whisk together the flour, baking soda, salt and sugar in a large bowl.
3. Cut in the cold butter into the dry ingredients. There should still be chunks of butter in the bread. It will melt into the dough as it bakes creating a tender crumb.

4. Add the buttermilk and stir until barely combined.
5. Turn the dough out onto a pastry mat or counter. (I didn't need more flour for the surface, but if your dough is extra sticky, lightly flour the surface.)
6. Knead 4-5 times just until all the flour gets combined and the mixture comes together. This should only take about 30 seconds.
7. Form the dough into a round loaf.
8. Place the loaf on the parchment paper.
9. Whisk together the buttermilk and melted butter. Brush this over the top of the dough.
10. Use a sharp knife to cut a cross on top of the dough.
11. Bake the loaf for 50 minutes. The internal temperature of the bread should be about 190-200°F.
12. Wrap in a tea towel while it is warm to soften the crust and to keep it soft.

28. Sage Butter Sauce
Prep Time: 5 Minutes

Cook Time: 20 minutes

Servings: 6

Ingredients

- 1 cup unsalted butter 2 sticks
- 14 fresh sage leaves
- 2 garlic cloves minced
- 2 tablespoons finely diced shallot

For Serving:

- 1 package butternut squash ravioli (or pasta, chicken or vegetables)

Instructions

1. If you're serving this ravioli, cook the ravioli according to package directions. While the ravioli is cooking, make the butter sage sauce.
2. Place a heavy bottomed saucepan on the stove.
3. Cut butter into 1 tablespoon chunks.
4. Place the butter in the saucepan and set stovetop to medium heat.
5. Allow the butter to melt, stirring often so that it melts evenly.
6. Once the butter is melted, set a timer for 5 minutes and allow the butter to simmer. Stir occasionally.
7. After 5 minutes, add the sage, minced garlic and diced shallot. Stir gently.

8. Allow this to simmer together for about 5 minutes.
    The sage will start to get crispy and the garlic & onion
    browned.
9. If you start to see little brown specks on the bottom of
    the pan, these are the milk solids. Don't stir the pan at
    this point.
10. After 5 minutes, remove the butter sauce from the
    heat and pour it into another bowl so it doesn't get too
    browned.
11. Drizzle the sauce over the cooked ravioli or other
    pasta, savory pumpkin dishes, chicken or vegetables.
    Add salt as needed.
12. It's also delicious served with crusty bread.

29. Homemade Lasagna
Prep Time: 30 Minutes

Cook Time: 2hrs 30 minutes

Servings: 15

Ingredients

- 1 pound sweet Italian sausage
- 1 pound ground chuck 80/20
- ½ cup diced onion
- 1 teaspoon minced garlic
- 28 ounces crushed tomatoes
- 12 ounces tomato paste
- 15 ounces tomato sauce
- ¼ cup water
- 2 tablespoons granulated sugar
- ½ cup freshly chopped basil
- ½ teaspoon fennel seeds
- 1 teaspoon Italian seasoning
- 1 teaspoon salt
- ¼ teaspoon black pepper
- 4 tablespoons chopped fresh parsley
- 12 lasagna noodles
- 15 ounces whole milk ricotta cheese
- 1 large egg
- dash nutmeg
- 1 pound whole milk mozzarella shredded
- 9-10 slices provolone cheese
- ½ cup freshly grated romano cheese
- ½ cup freshly grated parmesan cheese

Instructions

1. This makes a large pan of lasagna. I use a deep dish lasagna pan or a deep 9×13" baking dish.
2. In a large saucepan, cook the sausage, ground beef, onion and garlic until cooked through. Drain the fat.
3. Add the tomatoes, paste, sauce, water, sugar basil, fennel, Italian seasoning, salt, pepper and parsley. Stir well.
4. Simmer, covered, over low heat for 1 ½ hours, stirring occasionally.
5. Place the lasagna noodles in a pan of hot water and make certain they are completely covered. Allow them to sit for 30 minutes to soften, then drain the water.
6. In a small bowl, mix together the ricotta cheese, egg and nutmeg.
7. In a small bowl, mix together the Parmesan and Romano cheeses.

Let's Put Together The Lasagna!

1. Spread 1 ½ cups of meat sauce on the bottom of the lasagna pan.
2. Place 4 lasagna noodles over the sauce.
3. Spoon half of the ricotta mixture over the noodles.
4. Top with 2 cups of shredded mozzarella cheese.
5. Spread another 1 ½ cups of sauce over the mozzarella, then sprinkle with ⅓ cup of the Parmesan mixture.
6. Lay another 4 noodles over the cheese.
7. Top with the remaining ricotta mixture.
8. Lay 9-10 slices of provolone cheese over the ricotta, then top with 1 ½ cups meat sauce.
9. Sprinkle ⅓ cup Parmesan mixture over the sauce.

10. Top with 4 more noodles, the remaining sauce, 2 cups of mozzarella and the remaining Parmesan mixture.
11. Preheat the oven to 375°F. Bake immediately for 25 minutes (covered with foil) and then an additional 30 minutes with the foil removed.
12. Or…cover the unbaked casserole and refrigerate to save baking until the next day. If you choose to do this, remove the lasagna from the refrigerator 45 minutes before baking, then bake the same as above.
13. Allow the lasagna to cool for 15 minutes before slicing.
14. Store any leftovers in an airtight container in the fridge for up to 4 days.

30. Baked Brie with Hot Honey

Prep Time: 5 Minutes

Cook Time: 12 minutes

Servings: 6

Ingredients

Before Baking:

- 8 ounces double creme brie I used Alouette brand
- 1 tablespoon hot honey
- 2 cloves garlic finely diced
- ½ teaspoon red pepper flakes

After Baking:

- 1 tablespoon fresh thyme leaves
- 2 tablespoons chopped pistachios
- 2 tablespoons hot honey

Instructions

1. Preheat the oven to 350°F.
2. Place the brie wheel on a parchment lined baking sheet.
3. Slice 5 slices across the wheel of brie, going down about ¼" inch. Then turn the wheel and make an additional 5 slices across to make criss crosses.
4. Drizzle 1 tablespoon of honey over the top of the brie. Then sprinkle with ½ teaspoon red pepper flakes.

5. If the brie is at room temperature, bake for about 10 minutes. If it is right from the fridge, bake for 12-15 minutes.
6. Top the baked brie with the fresh thyme leaves, chopped pistachios, then drizzle with additional honey.
7. Serve alongside crusty bread, crackers, prosciutto and grapes.